Asian Keto Cookbook

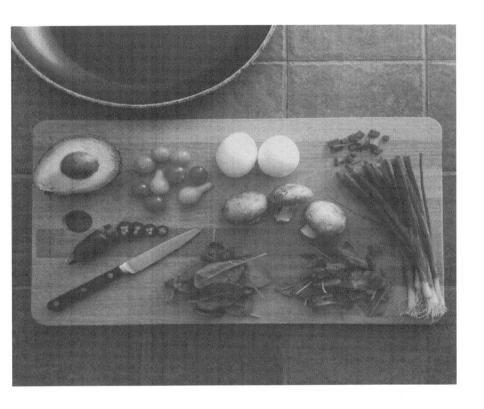

Created by:

Frankie Jepsen

Hello,

You're about to start a delicious new chapter in your Keto adventure! Good for you for making healthy choices. I hope you enjoy these delicious Asian dishes. Here are some exotic meals to get you inspired.

It may be beneficial to your health to follow your ketogenic lifestyle.

With limited options and ideas, going Asian-themed on a ketogenic diet appeared impossible. Now you can!

After trying out numerous dishes, we have chosen only the very best recipes to be covered in The Asian Keto Cookbook.

50+ Hand-picked, Asian Recipes – All of which are low-carb and will relate to your Keto goals

- Delicious Recipes from our tested kitchen- to yours
- Traditional Favorites — Classic dishes such as fried rice, stir-fry, soups, sauces, etc. made Keto and low-carb friendly
- Dairy-Free Recipes —Asian delicacies hardly ever include dairy and are terrific for those who are lactose intolerant
- Appetizers, Main Dishes and Desserts- All categories to keep you and your family satisfied
- Breaks Up the Typical Keto Menu —New and thrilling Asian flare that the Keto and low-carb way of life need to experience
- Multicultural Recipes - A wide range of Asian delicacies

Please contact me directly (555freshmail@gmail.com) with any suggestions or comments. A review on Amazon is apprciated; kindly enjoy this cookbook.

Thank you,

-FJ Jepsen

Appetizers

Asian Beef Salad

Beef Negimaki (Steak and Scallion Rolls)

Crispy Five Spice Wings

Spicy Roasted Broccoli

Low Carb Spring Rolls

Sweet and Spicy Brussels Sprouts

Sesame Chicken Bites

Tofu Lettuce Wraps

Japanese Cucumber Salad

Main Dishes

Singapore Stir Fry

Shrimp Chow Mein

Thai Coconut Chicken Soup

Chicken Peanut Pad Thai

Orange Beef

Cashew Beef Thai Stir Fry

Keto Asian Ground Beef

Asian Zucchini Noodles

Sweet and Sour Pork

Chicken and Cashews

Asian Glazed Salmon

Beef Cheeks

Sweet and Spicy Chicken

Keto Teriyaki Beef on a Stick

Asian Pho (Beef Noodle Soup)

Chinese BBQ Pork

Chinese Hot and Sour Soup

Meatball Asian Noodle Soup

Roasted Asian Salmon and Green Beans

Asian Shrimp and Brussels Sprouts Sheet Pan

Kung Pao Chicken

Shredded Beef Asian Style

Chicken Lo Mein

Asian Tuna Cakes

Broiled Asian Chicken Thighs

Meatballs in Coconut Broth

Thai Chicken Green Curry

Chicken with Satay Sauce

Thai Fish with Curry and Coconut

Almond Chili Beef and Cabbage Noodles

Sesame Crusted Chicken Tenders

Low Carb Asian Salmon Stir Fry

Miso Salmon with Cauliflower Rice

Fish with Japanese Mayo Sauce

Low Carb Pork Lo Mein

Desserts

Matcha Cheesecake

Coconut Almond Crisps

Matcha Pistachio Keto Mug Cake

Mango Panna Cotta

Japanese Cotton Cheesecake

Asian Beef Salad

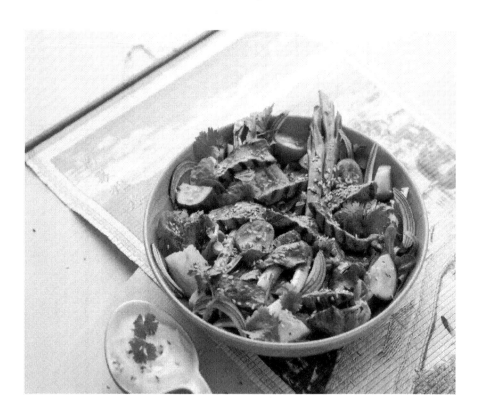

Cooking time: 5 minutes

Servings: 4

Ingredients:

- 1 lb. ribeye steak, sliced
- 4 scallions, chopped
- 6 oz cherry tomatoes, halved
- 4 oz cucumber, chopped
- 6 oz lettuce, chopped
- 1 onion, chopped
- 2 tablespoons sesame oil
- 2 tablespoons olive oil
- 2 tablespoons fish sauce
- 2 tablespoons fresh ginger, grated
- 2 teaspoons chili flakes
- 2 eggs yolk, room temperature
- 2 teaspoons Dijon mustard
- 1 cup avocado oil
- 1 tablespoon lime juice
- Salt, pepper, to taste
- Fresh cilantro, chopped

Instructions:

1. Mix mustard and egg yolks in a bowl. Slowly add avocado oil, whisking constantly. Add 2 tablespoons sesame oil, lime juice, salt and pepper. Mix well to combine.
2. Mix 2 tablespoons of olive oil, fish sauce, ginger and chili flakes in a bowl. Add the marinade to a Ziplock bag, add sliced beef. Marinate for about 15 minutes.
3. Preheat some oil in a skillet over medium heat. Add beef and cook for 3-4 minutes. Add scallions and cook for 1 minute more.
4. Add all the vegetables to a bowl, place the beef and scallions on top. Drizzle with mustard mixture.

Beef Negimaki
(Steak and Scallion Rolls)

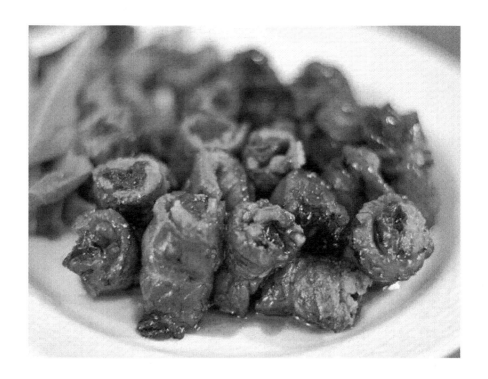

Cooking time: 10 minutes

Servings: 2

Ingredients:

- 2 bunches of scallions, trimmed
- 1 lb. flank steaks, pounded thinly
- 1 tablespoon coconut oil
- 1/3 cup tamari/soy sauce
- 1/3 cup rice wine vinegar
- 2 tablespoons fish sauce
- 1 teaspoon sesame oil
- 1 teaspoon Sriracha sauce
- 1 tablespoon ginger minced
- 1 garlic clove minced
- 2 tablespoons brown sugar

Instructions:

1. Mix tamari/soy sauce, vinegar, fish sauce, sesame oil, sriracha, ginger, garlic and sugar in a bowl.
2. Bring a small pot of water to a boil and add scallions. Cook for about 45 seconds.
3. Place about 5 scallions in the center of each pounded steak and roll up tightly.
4. Place the rolls in the marinade, let rest for about 1 hour.
5. Preheat oil in a pan over medium heat. Add rolls and cook for about 4-6 minutes, turning frequently.
6. Remove from pan and let rest for a couple of minutes before serving.

Crispy Five Spice Wings

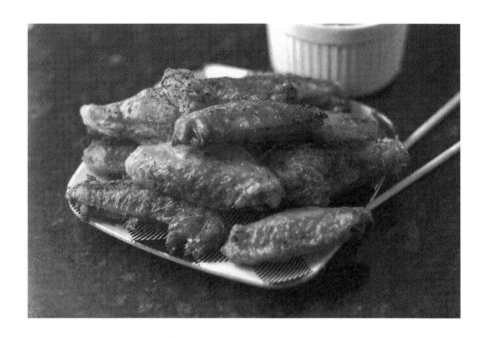

Cooking time: 30 minutes

Servings: 4

Ingredients:

- 1 ½ lbs. chicken wings
- 2 tablespoons avocado oil
- 2 tablespoons Chinese five spices
- 2 tablespoons ghee
- 1 jalapeno, sliced, for serving
- Salt, pepper, to taste

Instructions:

1. Preheat the oven to 400F. Line a baking sheet with foil.
2. Mix oil, spices, ghee, salt and pepper in a bowl. Pour into a Ziplock bag. Add wings and toss well to coat.
3. Place the wings on the baking sheet. Bake for 30 minutes.
4. Serve topped with sliced jalapeno.

Spicy Roasted Broccoli

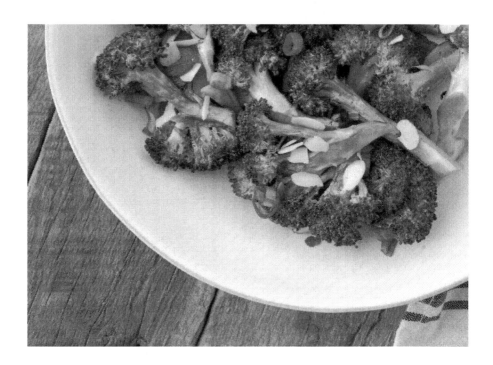

Cooking time: 10 minutes

Servings: 4

Ingredients:

- 4 cups broccoli florets, chopped
- ¼ cup mayonnaise
- 2 teaspoons Sriracha sauce
- 1 teaspoon soy sauce
- ½ teaspoon lime juice

Instructions:

1. Place broccoli florets in a heat proof dish and add about 2 tablespoons water. Microwave on high for 5 minutes.
2. Mix mayo, Sriracha, lime juice and soy sauce in a bowl. Add broccoli and toss well to coat.
3. Preheat a broiler and put the broccoli under the broiler for 3-4 minutes. Stir well and cook for another 2 minutes.

Low Carb Spring Rolls

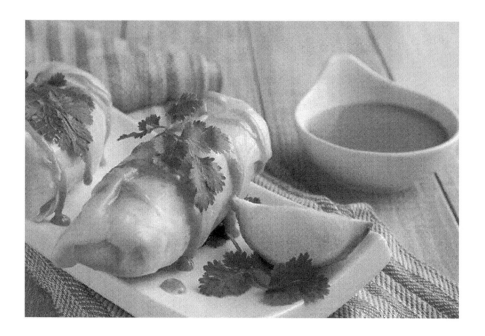

Cooking time: 20 minutes

Servings: 4

Ingredients:

- 3 quarts water
- 1 head green cabbage
- ¼ cup green onions, chopped
- 2 tablespoons parsley, chopped
- 2 garlic cloves, minced
- 1 tablespoon MCT oil
- 2 teaspoons of lime juice
- 1 teaspoon fresh ginger, grated
- ¼ teaspoon lime zest
- ½ pound ground chicken
- 1 tablespoon coconut oil
- Sea salt, black pepper, to taste

Instructions:

1. Add water and salt to a pot and bring to a boil.
2. Meanwhile, remove outer leaves from cabbage and make a cut through each cabbage leaf at the base where it attaches to the core. Shred the rest of the cabbage, for filling.
3. Add cabbage leaves to the pot with boiling water and cook for 1 minute. Remove from hot water and add to cold water for 1 minute.
4. Mix shredded cabbage, parsley, garlic, MCT oil, lime juice, ginger, lime zest, salt and pepper in a bowl. Toss well to coat.
5. Heat coconut oil in a skillet over medium heat. Add chicken and cook until no longer pink, for 6-8 minutes. Transfer the cooked chicken to a bowl with cabbage and marinate.
6. Place 1 cabbage leaf on your working surface and fill with the meat cabbage mixture. Fold tightly. Tie with a stem of cilantro or chives. Repeat with remaining leaves. Serve.

Sweet and Spicy Brussels sprouts

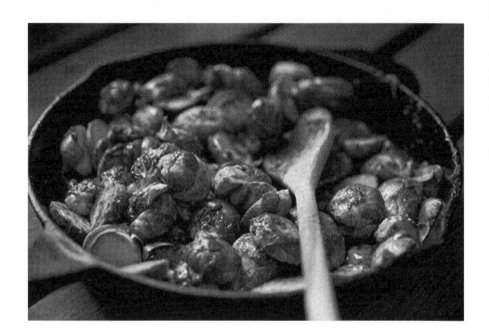

Cooking time: 5 minutes

Servings: 4

Ingredients:

- 1 lb. Brussels sprouts, trimmed and quartered
- 2 tablespoons sesame seed oil
- 1 tablespoon soy sauce
- 1 tablespoon Sriracha sauce
- 1 ½ tablespoons Sukrin Gold honey
- Pink Himalayan sea salt, to taste
- Ground black pepper, to taste
- Toasted sesame seeds, for serving
- Chopped green onions, for serving

Instructions:

1. Whisk sesame oil, soy sauce, Sriracha, honey, salt and black pepper in a bowl.
2. Add a little oil to a wok pan and preheat over medium heat. Add sprouts and cook for about 5 minutes, stirring occasionally.
3. Pour the sauce into the pan in the last 2 minutes of cooking, toss well until coated and remove from heat.
4. Serve topped with sesame seeds and onions.

Sesame Chicken Bites

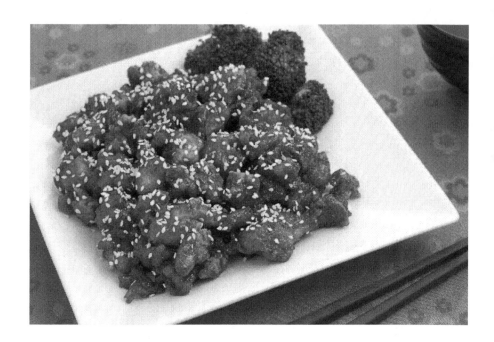

Cooking time: 15 minutes

Servings: 4

Ingredients:

- 2 lbs. chicken thighs, cut into bite-sized pieces
- 2 eggs
- 2 tablespoons cornstarch
- 2 tablespoons sesame oil + 2 tablespoons
- 4 tablespoons soy sauce
- 4 tablespoons Sukrin Gold honey
- 2 tablespoons vinegar
- ½ teaspoons xanthan gum
- 2 garlic cloves minced
- 1-inch piece of ginger, grated
- 4 tablespoons sesame seeds
- Salt, pepper, to taste

Instructions:

1. Whisk eggs and cornstarch in a bowl. Add chicken pieces, toss well to coat.
2. Preheat 2 tablespoons sesame oil in a skillet over medium heat. Add chicken and cook for about 10 minutes, stirring often.
3. Meanwhile, mix soy sauce, honey, vinegar, xanthan gum, garlic, ginger, 2 tablespoons sesame oil, sesame seeds, salt and pepper in a bowl.
4. Pour the sesame sauce into the skillet with the chicken. Cook for an additional 5 minutes.
5. Serve with sesame seeds and green onions.

Tofu Lettuce Wraps

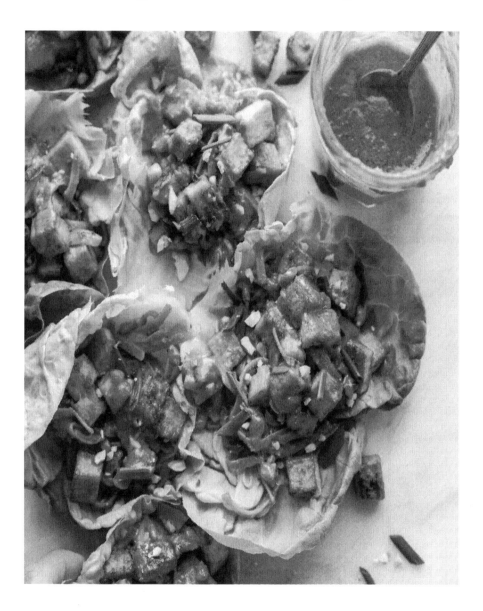

Cooking time: 15 minutes

Servings: 4

Ingredients:

- 1 package (14 oz) extra-firm tofu
- 8 large inner leaves of romaine lettuce
- 8 oz baby mushrooms, chopped
- 1 can (8 oz) water chestnuts, drained and chopped
- 2 garlic cloves minced
- 2 teaspoons fresh ginger, grated
- 4 green onions, sliced
- 3 tablespoons hoisin sauce
- 3 tablespoons soy sauce
- 2 tablespoons rice vinegar
- 1 teaspoon sesame oil
- 2 teaspoons canola oil
- ¼ teaspoon red pepper flakes

Instructions:

1. Mix hoisin, soy sauce, rice vinegar, and sesame oil in a bowl. Press the tofu and squeeze out as much liquid as possible. Crumble the tofu.
2. Heat canola oil in a large skillet over medium heat. Add tofu and cook for about 5 minutes. Add mushrooms and cook for about 3 minutes more.
3. Add water chestnuts, garlic, ginger, red pepper flakes, and half of the green onions, cook for 30 more seconds.
4. Add the sauce to the skillet and stir well to coat. Cook for about 1 minute.
5. Add tofu mixture on top of each lettuce leaf. Top with the remaining green onions and serve.

Cucumber Sushi Rolls

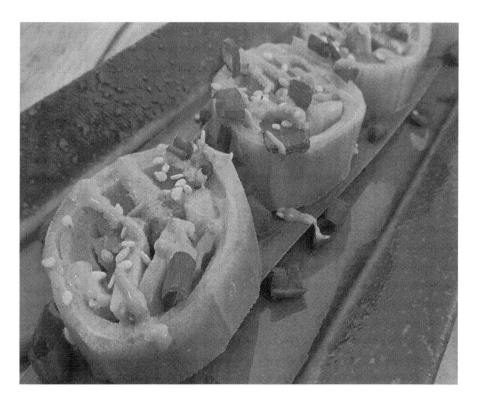

Cooking time: 5 minutes

Servings: 2

Ingredients:

- 2 cucumbers, peeled, ends trimmed
- ½ lb. Tuna steak, chopped
- 8 shrimp, chopped
- ½ avocado, chopped
- 2 tablespoons mayonnaise
- 2 teaspoons Sriracha
- 1 stalk green onion, chopped
- ½ teaspoon sesame seeds

Instructions:

1. Using a long, wet and sharp knife, hollow out the cucumbers.
2. Mix tuna, shrimp, avocado, sriracha and mayo in a bowl. Fill each cucumber with the mixture.
3. Slice the stuffed cucumber into rolls and serve topped with sesame seeds and additional mayo.

Japanese Cucumber Salad

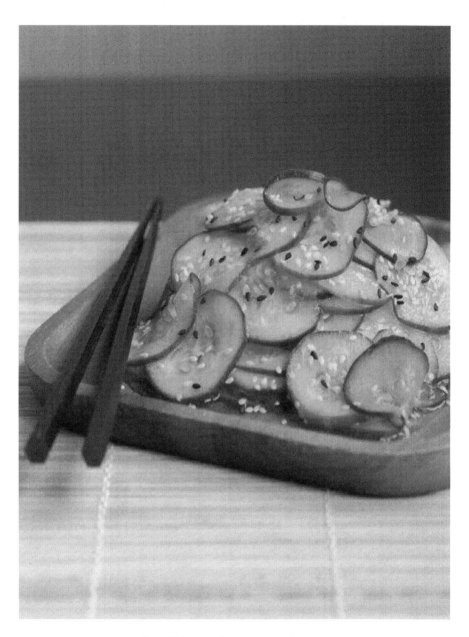

Cooking time: 5 minutes

Servings: 2

Ingredients:

- 2 Japanese or Persian cucumbers, peeled
- 1 teaspoon sesame seeds
- 2 tablespoons rice vinegar
- 3 ½ teaspoons sweetener of choice
- ½ teaspoon soy sauce
- 1 tablespoon dried seaweed
- Salt, to taste

Instructions:

1. Soak seaweed in water for about 5 minutes. Drain and squeeze out excess liquid.
2. Mix rice vinegar, soy sauce, sweetener and sesame seeds in a bowl.
3. Rub the cucumbers with salt and slice them. Add the slices to a bowl, top with seaweed.
4. Serve sliced cucumbers with the sauce. Toss well to coat.

Singapore Stir Fry

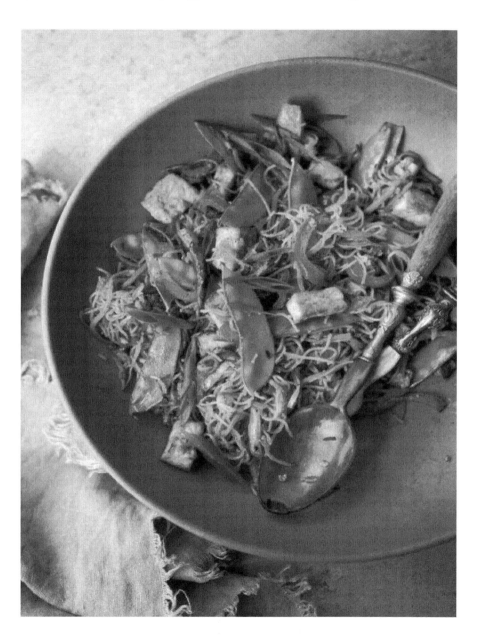

Cooking time: 10 minutes

Servings: 2

Ingredients:

- 5 oz chicken thighs, sliced
- 1 bunch Bok Choy, sliced
- 2 oz bean sprouts
- 3 oz shrimp (prawns), cooked, chopped
- 1 onion, sliced
- 1 celery stick, sliced
- 1 garlic clove, chopped
- 1 packet angel hair Konjac Noodles
- 2 slices bacon, thinly sliced
- 1 tablespoon sesame oil
- 2 teaspoons of curry powder
- 2 tablespoons soy sauce

Instructions:

1. Add noodles to a colander and run hot water over them for 3 minutes. Drain and set aside.
2. Preheat oil in a skillet over medium heat. Add bacon and cook for 1 minute. Add chicken and cook for 2-3 minutes, until brown.
3. Add onion and garlic and cook for 2 additional minutes. Add celery, shrimp and curry powder, stir well to combine.
4. Add drained noodles to skillet and stir all the ingredients to combine. Sauté for 2 minutes.
5. Add soy sauce, bok choy and bean sprouts; toss well to cover all the ingredients in sauce.
6. Cook for 1-2 minutes and remove from heat. Serve hot.

Shrimp Chow Mein

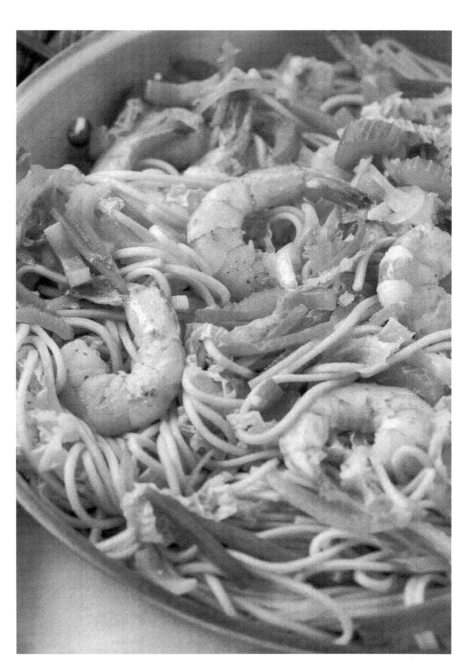

Cooking time: 1 hour

Servings: 4

Ingredients:

- 1 spaghetti squash, halved lengthwise
- ¾ lb. shrimp, peeled and deveined
- 4 cups Coleslaw mix
- 2 green onions, sliced
- 2 garlic cloves minced
- 2 dried red peppers
- ¼ teaspoon fresh ginger minced
- 10 peppercorns
- 1 tablespoon sesame oil
- 2 tablespoons coconut amino
- A pinch of sea salt

Instructions:

1. Preheat the oven to 375F. Bake the squash for 45-50 minutes. Remove from the oven and shred with a fork.
2. Mix garlic, ginger, green onion, red peppers and peppercorns in a bowl. Preheat the sesame oil in a pan over medium heat and add the garlic ginger mix. Cook for about 1 minute.
3. Add shrimp and cook until pink on all sides, stirring frequently.
4. Add slaw mix and cook for 1-2 minutes. Add the squash spaghetti and stir well to combine.
5. Add coconut amino and toss well to coat. Add salt, stir well and serve.

Thai Coconut Chicken Soup

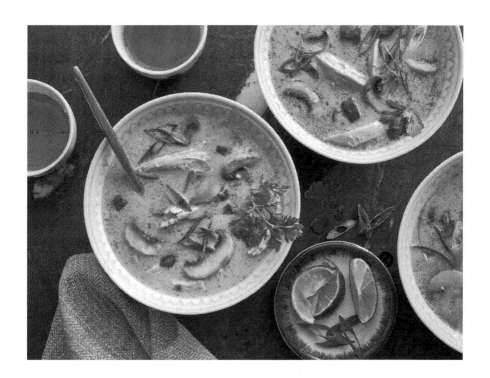

Cooking time: 45 minutes

Servings: 4

Ingredients:

- 1 lb. chicken thighs, boneless skinless
- 6 cups chicken broth
- 2 stalks lemongrass, cut into about 4 1-inch pieces
- 1 lime, juiced and zested
- 1-inch fresh ginger, grated
- 10 oz mushrooms, chopped
- 1 ½ cups coconut cream
- 1 tablespoon fish sauce
- 1 chili pepper
- Fresh cilantro, chopped, for serving
- Sea salt, to taste

Instructions:

1. Add chicken broth to a pan and heat it over medium heat. Add lemongrass, lime juice and zest, ginger and salt.
2. Bring the broth to a boil and let simmer for 20 minutes. Strain.
3. Add chicken and mushrooms to the strained broth. Cook for 20 minutes.
4. Remove chicken thighs from the broth and shred. Return to the pot. Add coconut cream and fish sauce.
5. Let the soup cool for about 15 minutes. Serve topped with chili peppers and cilantro.

Chicken Peanut Pad Thai

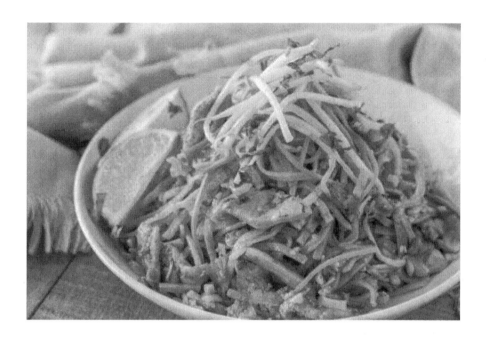

Cooking time: 15 minutes

Servings: 4

Ingredients:

- 16 oz chicken thighs, boneless skinless
- 1 oz peanuts
- 1 tablespoon olive oil
- 1 white onion, chopped
- 2 garlic cloves minced
- 2 large zucchinis, spiralized into noodles
- 1 egg
- 2 tablespoons soy sauce
- 1 lime
- ½ teaspoon chili flakes
- Salt, pepper, to taste

Instructions:

1. Preheat oil in a skillet over medium heat. Add onions and cook for about 3 minutes.
2. Season chicken with salt and pepper, add to the skillet. Cook for about 5-7 minutes on each side.
3. Remove chicken from skillet and shred with a fork. Crack an egg in the center of the skillet. Cook for a few seconds and then scramble it into large chunks.
4. Add zoodles to the pan and cook for 2 minutes, tossing continuously.
5. Add chicken, soy sauce, lime juice and chili flakes. Stir well to combine all the ingredients.
6. Serve chicken topped with peanuts and lime.

Orange Beef

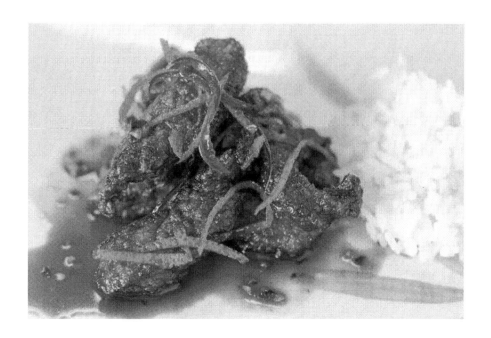

Cooking time: 15 minutes

Servings: 4

Ingredients:

- 1 lb. beef top sirloin, cut into strips
- ¼ cup low-sodium soy sauce
- ¼ cup water
- 1 tablespoon honey
- ¼ teaspoon red pepper flakes
- 2 tablespoons butter
- 2 green onions, thinly sliced
- 1 tablespoon fresh ginger root, minced
- 1 tablespoon orange zest, cut into thin strips
- 2 garlic cloves, crushed
- ½ teaspoon xanthan gum
- 1 tablespoon rice vinegar

Instructions:

1. Mix soy sauce, water, honey and red pepper flakes in a bowl. Pat dry beef slices with paper towels.
2. Preheat 1 tablespoon butter in a skillet over medium heat. Add beef and brown on all sides. Transfer to a plate.
3. Add the remaining butter to the skillet and add green onions, ginger and orange zest. Cook for 1-2 minutes. Add garlic and xanthan gum and cook for 30 seconds more.
4. Add rice vinegar, stir well and deglaze the pan. Cook for 1-2 minutes and add soy sauce honey mixture. Simmer until sauce thickens. Serve topped with more green onions.

Cashew Beef Thai Stir Fry

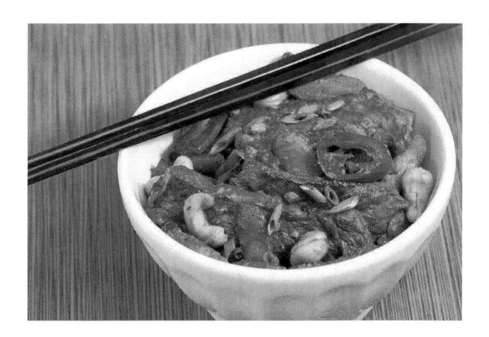

Cooking time: 20 minutes

Servings: 2

Ingredients:

- 1 lb. beef, sliced
- 2 garlic cloves, minced
- 1 teaspoon fresh ginger, minced
- 1 carrot, sliced
- ½ red onion, sliced
- 1 zucchini, chopped
- 1 jalapeno, sliced
- ¼ cup beef broth
- ¼ cup coconut milk
- 1 oz cashews
- 1 bunch fresh basil
- 2 tablespoons toasted sesame seed oil
- ¼ teaspoon red pepper flakes
- ¼ teaspoon Chinese Five Spice
- Salt, pepper, to taste

Instructions:

1. Preheat oil in a skillet over medium heat. Add garlic, onion, ginger and carrots and cook for about 3-4 minutes.
2. Add zucchini and jalapeno, also add red pepper flakes, Five Spice, salt and pepper. Stir well to combine, cook for 2-3 minutes. Transfer to a plate.
3. Add more oil to the skillet and add beef. Cook until browned on all sides.
4. Add vegetables back to the skillet. Add broth and coconut milk. Add cashews and cover the skillet, cook for 8 minutes.
5. Add fresh basil and stir to combine. Cook for 5 minutes and serve.

Keto Asian Ground Beef

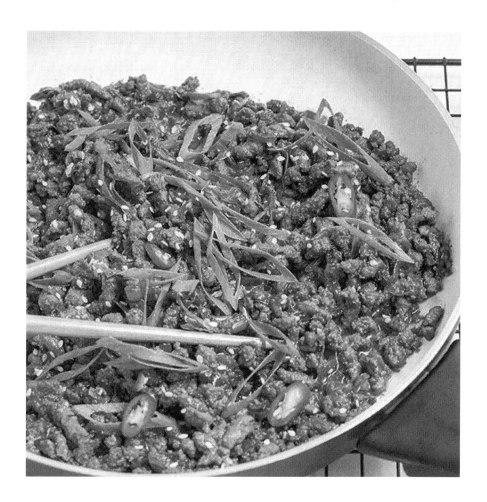

Cooking time: 15 minutes

Servings: 4

Ingredients:

- 1 lb. ground beef
- 4 tablespoons sesame oil
- 2 garlic cloves, crushed
- 2 small red chilies, thinly sliced
- 1 onion, thinly sliced
- ¼ cup scallions, sliced
- 1 teaspoon sesame seeds
- ¼ cup tamari sauce
- 2 tablespoons sweetener of choice
- ½ teaspoon fresh ginger, grated

Instructions:

1. Mix 2 tablespoons sesame oil, tamari, sweetener and ginger in a bowl.
2. Preheat 2 tablespoons of oil in a skillet over medium heat. Add garlic, scallions, chili and onion and cook for 2-3 minutes.
3. Add beef and cook for 7-8 minutes until browned.
4. Pour the tamari ginger sauce over the meat and simmer until the sauce has thickened, stirring frequently to coat the beef.

Asian Zucchini Noodles

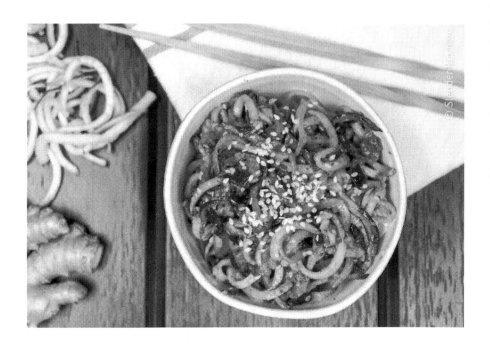

Cooking time: 10 minutes

Servings: 2

Ingredients:

- 2 zucchinis, spiralized
- ¼ cup dark soy sauce
- 1 teaspoon Sriracha sauce
- 1 tablespoon dark brown sugar
- 1 teaspoon olive or sesame oil
- ¼ cup onion minced
- 2 garlic cloves minced

Instructions:

1. Whisk together soy sauce, Sriracha and sugar in a bowl.
2. Preheat oil in a skillet over medium heat. Add onions and cook for 2 minutes. Add garlic and cook for 30 seconds more.
3. Add the sauce to the skillet, cook for 1 minute and add the zucchini noodles. Cook for 1-2 minutes, stirring frequently to coat the noodles with sauce. Serve!

Sweet and Sour Pork

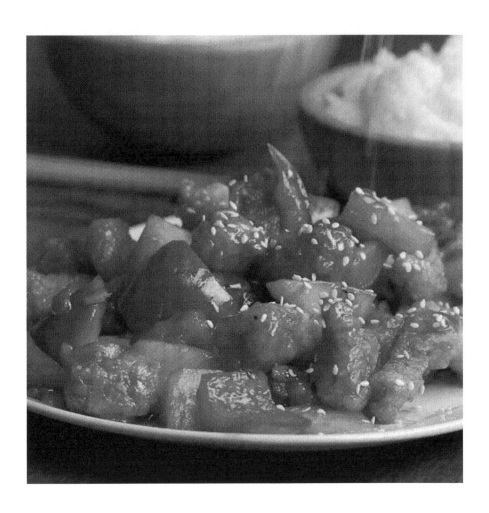

Cooking time: 25 minutes

Servings: 2

Ingredients:

- 1 lb. pork fillet, sliced
- ⅓ cup almond flour
- 2 tablespoons protein powder
- 1 teaspoon baking powder
- 1 egg
- 2 tablespoons chilled sparkling water
- 2 teaspoons of sesame oil
- ½ bell pepper, diced
- 2 scallions, sliced
- 2 teaspoons sesame seeds
- Salt, to taste

For Sweet and Sour Sauce:

- ⅓ cup rice wine vinegar
- ⅓ cup honey
- ¼ cup tomato sauce
- ¼ cup water
- 1 tablespoon tamari sauce
- 1 teaspoon garlic powder
- ½ teaspoon xanthan gum

Instructions:

1. First cook the sauce. Add wine vinegar, honey, tomato sauce, tamari sauce and garlic powder to a frying pan and heat over medium heat. Add xanthan gum and bring everything to a simmer. Cook until the sauce has thickened and remove from heat.
2. Heat the deep fryer oil to 355F. Mix almond flour, protein powder, baking powder and salt in a bowl.
3. Add egg and sparkling water and whisk until a thick batter is formed.
4. Dip the pork strips into the batter and then slowly drop into the hot oil. Cook until browned, then flip over and cook for 2-3 minutes.
5. Preheat oil in a skillet over medium heat. Add onion and pepper and cook for 5-8 minutes.

6. Reduce the heat to low and add the cooked sauce. Heat for 1 minute. Add crispy pork strips to the pan and toss well to coat with sauce.
7. Serve topped with scallions and sesame seeds.

Chicken and Cashews

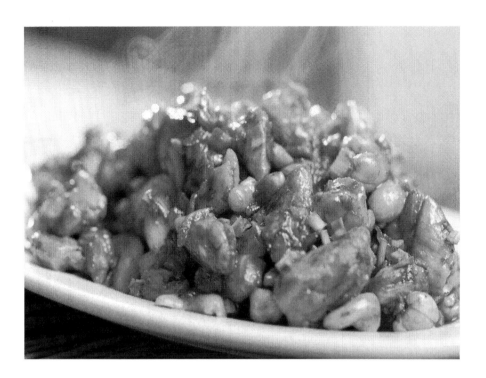

Cooking time: 20 minutes

Servings: 4

Ingredients:

- 1 lb. chicken breast, skinless boneless, cubed
- 1 cup cashews, toasted
- ½ onion, sliced
- 2 tablespoons green onions, chopped
- 1 garlic clove, crushed
- 2 teaspoons xanthan gum
- 2 teaspoons dry sherry
- ½ teaspoon of ginger root, grated
- 2 tablespoons dark soy sauce
- 2 tablespoons hoisin sauce
- 1 teaspoon sweetener of choice
- 2 tablespoons water
- 4 tablespoons peanut oil
- 1 teaspoon sesame seed oil

Instructions:

1. Add chicken to a bowl, add xanthan gum, sherry and ginger, stir well to combine.
2. Mix soy sauce, hoisin sauce, sweetener and 2 tablespoons water in a separate bowl, stir until smooth.
3. Preheat oil in a skillet or a wok pan over medium heat. Add garlic and onion, cook for about 30 seconds. Add chicken and cook for 1-2 minutes, stirring. Discard the garlic from the pan and reduce the heat to low.
4. Add the soy sauce mixture, cook for 1-2 minutes. Add cashews and stir for 30 seconds.
5. Serve topped with sesame seeds and green onions.

Asian Glazed Salmon

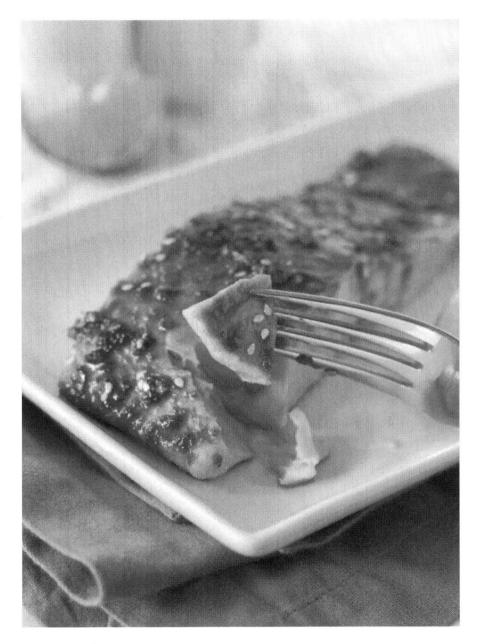

Cooking time: 20 minutes

Servings: 6

Ingredients:

- 6 salmon fillets
- ½ cup liquid amino
- 1 teaspoon chili paste (Sambal)
- ½ cup Swerve sweetener
- 2 tablespoons rice vinegar
- 2 teaspoons toasted sesame oil
- 2 teaspoons fresh ginger, grated
- 1 teaspoon garlic, grated
- ½ lime, juiced
- Sesame seeds, for serving

Instructions:

1. Preheat the oven to 400F.
2. Mix amino, chili paste, Swerve, vinegar, sesame oil, ginger, garlic and lime juice in a bowl. Add the mixture to the pan and preheat over medium heat. Simmer until thick.
3. Place the salmon fillets on a baking rack skin side down. Brush each fillet with the glaze from all sides and cook for 10 minutes.
4. Remove from the oven and increase the heat to 450F. Brush salmon fillets with extra glaze and cook for 3-5 minutes.
5. Serve topped with sesame seeds.

Beef Cheeks

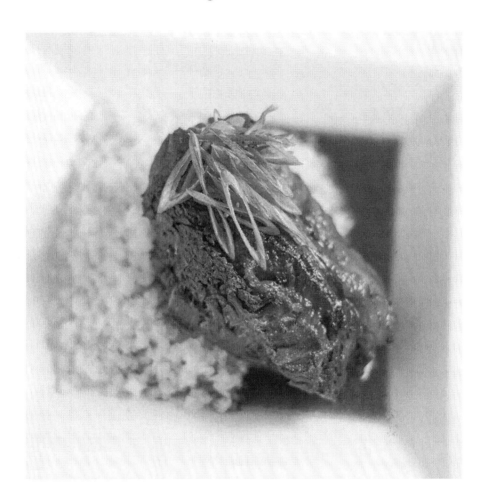

Cooking time: 1 hour 5 minutes

Servings: 4

Ingredients:

- 2 lbs. beef cheeks, cut into big pieces
- 1 orange, zested
- 2 scallions, sliced
- 3 garlic cloves, sliced
- 2-inch piece fresh ginger, sliced
- ½ cup Chinese cooking wine
- 1 cup tamari sauce
- 1/3 cup Sukrin Gold
- 1 tablespoon sesame oil
- 3 anise stars
- 1 cinnamon stick

Instructions:

1. Preheat oil in a large saucepan over medium heat. Add orange zest, scallions, garlic, ginger, cooking wine, tamari, sukrin gold, sesame oil, anise and cinnamon, stir well to combine. Simmer for 2-3 minutes.
2. Add beef and stir well to coat with sauce. Reduce the heat to low and cover the pan.
3. Cook for 1 hour on low heat. Serve.

Sweet and Spicy Chicken

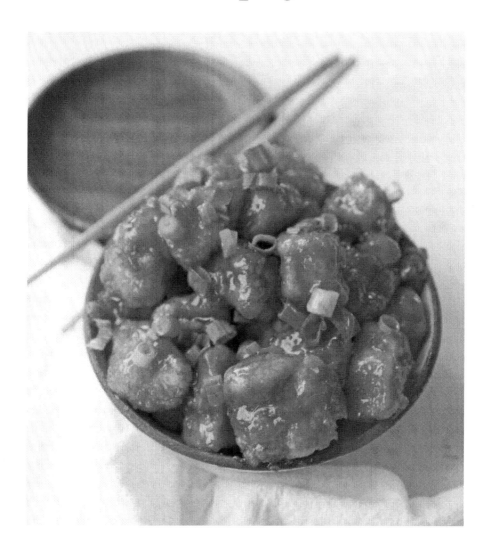

Cooking time: 40 minutes

Servings: 4

Ingredients:

- 1 lb. chicken thighs, boneless skinless
- 1 lb. chicken breast, boneless skinless
- 3 tablespoons low sodium soy sauce + 2 teaspoons
- ¾ teaspoons Stevia
- 2 tablespoons garlic chili paste + 2 teaspoons
- 1 garlic clove, minced
- 2 teaspoons ginger, minced

Instructions:

1. Mix soy sauce, Stevia, chili garlic paste, garlic, and ginger in the saucepan and preheat over medium heat.
2. Add chicken and stir well to coat. Cover the pan.
3. Cook over low heat for 25-30 minutes. Remove the chicken from the pan and transfer to a plate.
4. Bring the sauce to a boil and cook for 8-10 minutes until it thickens. Serve chicken with the sauce.

Keto Teriyaki Beef on a Stick

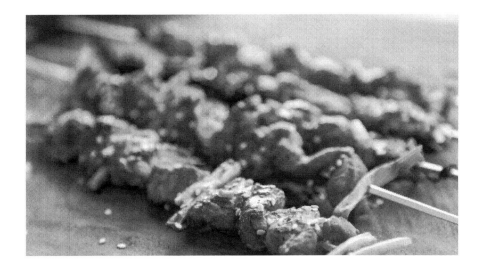

Cooking time: 10 minutes

Servings: 4

Ingredients:

- 1 lb. lean beef, cubed
- 2 tablespoons soy sauce
- 2 tablespoons rice wine vinegar
- 2 tablespoons erythritol
- 1 teaspoon sesame oil
- 1 teaspoon avocado oil

Instructions:

1. Mix sesame oil, avocado oil, soy sauce, rice wine vinegar, and erythritol in a bowl. Add beef and toss well to coat meat with the sauce. Let marinate for at least 1 hour.
2. Remove beef from the refrigerator 30 minutes before cooking. Preheat the grill to medium high. Alternatively, you can cook beef on a skillet or in the oven.
3. Thread the meat onto skewers. Grill for 2-3 minutes per side.
4. Add sauce to a pan and cook over medium heat for 2-3 minutes. Serve skewers topped with the sauce.

Asian Pho (Beef Noodle Soup)

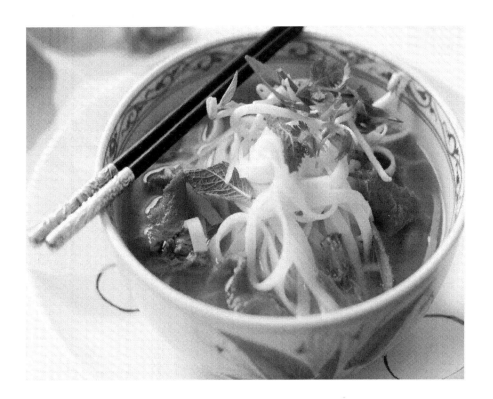

Cooking time: 30 minutes

Servings: 4

Ingredients:

- 6 cups beef broth
- ½ lb. sirloin steak
- 16 oz shirataki noodles, rinsed
- 2 onions, quartered
- 1 (4-inch) piece ginger, peeled and quartered
- 2 cinnamon sticks
- 2 teaspoons whole coriander seeds
- 1 tablespoon soy sauce
- 1 tablespoon fish sauce
- 2 scallions, sliced
- ¼ cup fresh cilantro leaves, chopped
- 1 lime, quartered

Instructions:

1. Mix broth, onions, ginger, cinnamon sticks, coriander seeds, soy sauce and fish sauce in a saucepan. Bring to a boil over high heat, then reduce the heat to low. Cover the pan and cook for 30 minutes.
2. Put the beef on a plate and cover with plastic wrap. Freeze for 15 minutes. Remove the beef from the freezer and slice with a sharp knife.
3. Add noodles to a colander and rinse with warm water. Strain the broth and return to the pan.
4. While the broth is simmering, put the beef on a plate, cover with plastic wrap, and freeze for 15 minutes. The edges of the beef should feel firm to the touch, but the beef should not be frozen through.
5. Divide noodles and beef slices among serving bowls and top with hot broth. Add lime juice, serve topped with scallions and cilantro.

Chinese BBQ Pork

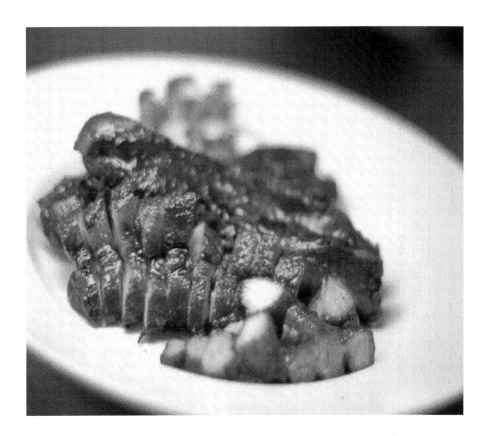

Cooking time: 45 minutes

Servings: 6

Ingredients:

- 2 lbs. pork butt, cut into large pieces
- ¼ cup low carb sweet soy sauce
- 2 teaspoon sesame oil
- 1 teaspoon garlic powder
- 1 teaspoon Chinese Five Spice

Instructions:

1. Mix soy sauce, sesame oil, garlic and five spice in a bowl.
2. Add pork pieces to a deep dish and pour half of the sauce on top. Coat the meat with the sauce. Cover and marinate in the fridge overnight. Store the remaining marinade in the fridge too.
3. Preheat the oven to 390F. Line a baking tray with foil and place the beef pieces on the tray.
4. Cook for 10 minutes, then brush with more marinade from all sides and turn. Cook for another 10 minutes and turn again, brush with marinade. Cook for the final 15-20 minutes.
5. Let rest for 10 minutes before serving.

Chinese Hot and Sour Soup

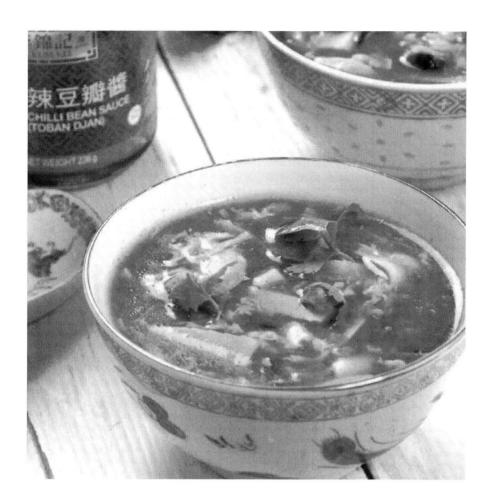

Cooking time: 50 minutes

Servings: 4

Ingredients:

- 1 lb. chicken breast, cubed
- 8 ½ cups water
- ½ onion
- 1 oz dried shiitake mushrooms
- 1 jar bamboo shoots, sliced
- 1 bell pepper, sliced
- 1 carrot, sliced
- 2 eggs, beaten
- 1 chili pepper, chopped
- 1 piece (1-inch) fresh ginger, whole
- 1-piece ginger, chopped
- 1 garlic clove, chopped
- 4 tablespoons soy sauce
- 5 tablespoons rice vinegar
- 1 teaspoon white pepper
- 2 teaspoons paprika powder
- 2 teaspoons xanthan gum
- Green onions, chopped, for serving
- Salt, to taste

Instructions:

1. Soak mushrooms in water for 30-60 minutes.
2. Add water to a saucepan, add chicken, whole piece ginger and onion, bring to a boil. Cook for 35-45 minutes.
3. Add chili, chopped ginger, salt and garlic to a mortar and pestle until smooth.
4. Remove the onion and ginger from the broth. Add chopped vegetables to the pan. Add chili paste, rice vinegar, soy sauce, white pepper and paprika. Stir well to combine. Season with salt. Cook for 10-15 minutes.
5. Pour beaten eggs to the soup stirring all the time. Let simmer for 1-2 minutes.
6. Add xanthan gum and let simmer until thick. Serve soup topped with green onions.

Meatball Asian Noodle Soup

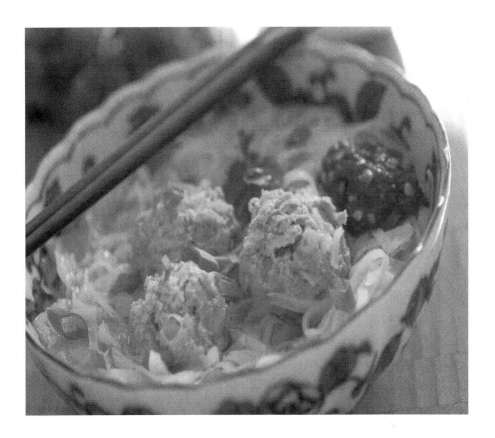

Cooking time: 30 minutes

Servings: 4

Ingredients:

- 3 cups shirataki noodles, drained and rinsed
- 2 cups cabbage, shredded
- ¼ cup radish, cut into thin strips
- ¼ cup carrot, shredded
- ½ cup scallions, chopped
- ½ cup fresh cilantro, chopped
- 1 teaspoon sesame oil
- 2 tablespoons ginger minced
- 1 teaspoon garlic, minced
- 4 cups chicken broth
- 2 cups of water.
- 1 tablespoon soy sauce
- 1 tablespoon fish sauce
- ½ teaspoon of red pepper flakes
- Salt, to taste
- 1 lime, cut into wedges

For Meatballs:

- 1 lb. ground turkey
- 1 egg
- 1/3 cup almond flour
- 1 teaspoon ginger minced
- 1/3 cup scallions, chopped
- 1 tablespoon soy sauce
- ½ teaspoon garlic powder
- Salt, to taste

Instructions:

1. Preheat the oven to 375F. Line a baking tray with parchment paper.
2. Mix ground turkey, egg, almond flour, ginger, scallions, soy sauce, garlic powder and salt in a bowl. Form the mixture into medium sized balls and place them on the baking tray. Cook for 12 minutes.

3. Heat sesame oil in a saucepan over medium heat. Add minced garlic and ginger and cook for 1 minute. Add broth, water, soy sauce, fish sauce, red pepper flakes and salt and bring everything to a boil. Cook for 10 minutes. Strain the broth and return to the pan.
4. Add shirataki noodles, meatballs, cabbage, radish, carrot, scallions and cilantro to a large pot. Pour hot broth on top and stir well to combine everything. Serve with lime wedges.

Roasted Asian Salmon and Green Beans

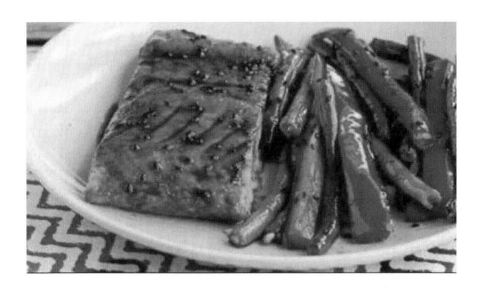

Cooking time: 20 minutes

Servings: 4

Ingredients:

- 4 salmon fillets, skinless
- 1 lb. fresh green beans, ends trimmed
- 1 bell pepper, sliced
- 2 teaspoons peanut oil

For the Glaze:
- 1/3 cup soy sauce
- 2 tablespoons rice vinegar
- 2 tablespoons of sweeteners of choice
- 1 tablespoon sesame oil
- ½ teaspoon garlic powder
- Salt, to taste

Instructions:

1. Preheat the oven to 400F. Spray baking sheet with cooking spray.
2. Mix soy sauce, rice vinegar, sweetener, sesame oil, and garlic powder in a bowl.
3. Add beans and bell pepper to the tray and brush with peanut oil. Season everything with salt.
4. Cook for 10 minutes. Place salmon fillets on the baking tray on top of veggies and brush each fillet with the glaze, from all sides.
5. Cook for 10-12 minutes. Remove from the oven and brush the salmon and vegetables with the remaining glaze. Serve hot.

Asian Shrimp and Brussels Sprouts Sheet Pan

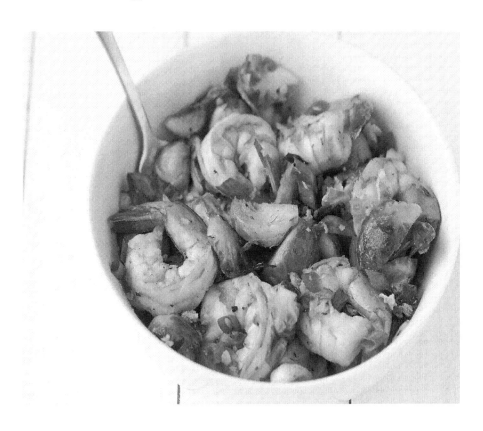

Cooking time: 25 minutes

Servings: 4

Ingredients:

- 1 lb. frozen shrimp, thawed and drained
- 1 lb. Brussels sprouts, trimmed and halved
- 2 tablespoons olive oil
- 1/3 cup soy sauce
- 2 tablespoons rice vinegar
- 2 tablespoons sweetener of choice
- 2 teaspoons agave nectar
- 1 tablespoon sesame oil
- ½ teaspoon garlic powder
- Salt, pepper, to taste

Instructions:

1. Mix soy sauce, vinegar, sweetener, agave nectar, sesame oil and garlic powder in a bowl.
2. Preheat the oven to 400F. Spay a baking sheet with cooking spray. Pat dry shrimp with paper towels.
3. Add shrimp to marinade mixture and toss well to coat. Let rest for about 10 minutes.
4. Drizzle sprouts with olive oil, salt and pepper. Spread on a baking tray in one layer. Cook for 15 minutes.
5. Remove sprouts from the oven and tops with shrimps. Bake for 6-8 minutes.
6. Stir cooked sprouts and shrimp, brush with the remaining marinade.

Kung Pao Chicken

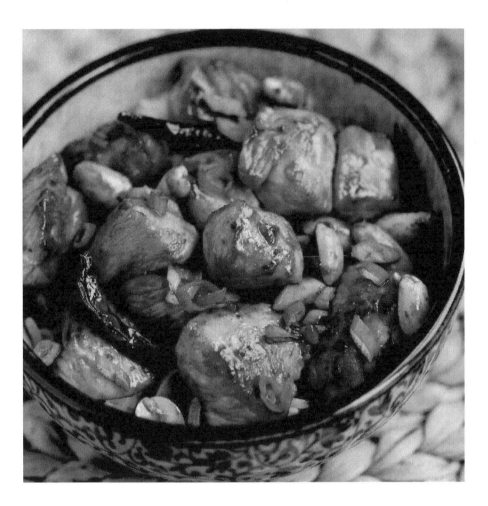

Cooking time: 12 minutes

Servings: 4

Ingredients:

- ¾ lb. Chicken thighs, cut into 1-inch pieces
- 1 bell pepper, chopped
- 1 zucchini, chopped
- 2 dried red chili peppers
- 3 tablespoons olive oil
- 2/3 cup roasted cashews
- ¼ teaspoon xanthan gum
- 3 tablespoons coconut amino
- 1 teaspoon fish sauce
- 2 teaspoons of sesame oil
- 1 teaspoon apple cider vinegar
- ½ teaspoon red pepper chili flakes
- ½ teaspoon fresh ginger minced
- 2 garlic cloves minced
- 2 tablespoons water
- 2 teaspoons erythritol
- Salt, black pepper, to taste

Instructions:

1. Mix coconut amino, fish sauce, sesame oil, vinegar, chili flakes, ginger, garlic, water and sweetener in a bowl.
2. Season chicken with salt, pepper and 1 tablespoon of the sauce mixture.
3. Preheat oil in a skillet over medium heat. Cook chicken for 5-6 minutes, stirring occasionally.
4. Add zucchini, bell peppers and dried chili peppers, cook for 2-3 minutes more. Add the remaining sauce mixture and add xanthan gum and cashews. Stir well to combine all the ingredients. Increase heat to high.
5. Cook until the sauce thickens, season with salt and pepper. Remove from heat and serve over zucchini "noodles" or cauliflower rice.

Shredded Beef Asian Style

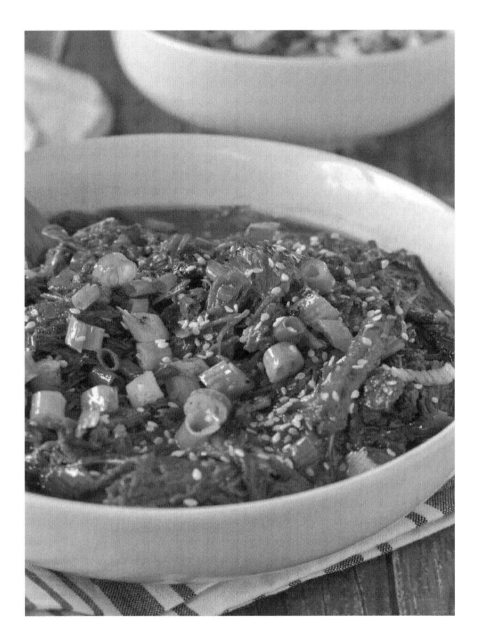

Cooking time: 45 minutes

Servings: 5

Ingredients:

- 2 lbs. beef chuck roast, cut into bite-sized pieces
- 1 cup beef stock
- 3 garlic cloves, sliced
- 2 tablespoons ginger, chopped
- 1 red chili, sliced
- 2 tablespoons sesame oil
- ½ cup hoisin sauce
- 1/3 cup tamari sauce
- 1 teaspoon Chinese Five Spice
- 1 teaspoon black pepper

Instructions:

1. Mix sesame oil, garlic, ginger and chili in a pan, sauté for 2 minutes.
2. Add hoisin sauce, tamari, Five Spice and pepper, stir well to combine. Add beef and coat with sauce. Cook for 5-6 minutes.
3. Add beef stock, making sure the beef is covered. Bring to a boil and reduce the heat to low, cover the lid.
4. Cook for 25-30 minutes. Remove the beef from the pan and shred. Cook the sauce until thick.
5. Return the beef to the pot and serve hot.
6. **NOTE.** If you want the beef to be crispy just fry it before serving.

This is a nice variation, you can make it crispy or a softer texture. It is entirely up to you!

Chicken Lo Mein

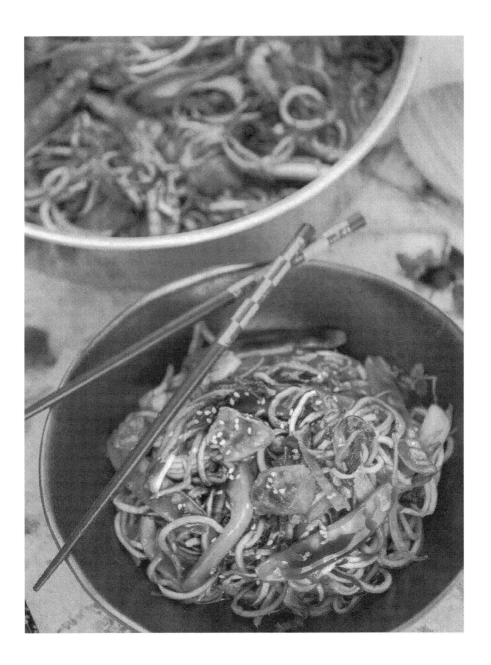

Cooking time: 15 minutes

Servings: 4

Ingredients:

- 1 lb. chicken breast, sliced
- 2 zucchinis, spiralized
- 2 tablespoons dry sherry
- 1/3 cup coconut amino
- 2 garlic cloves minced
- 1 tablespoon fresh ginger, grated
- 2 tablespoons coconut oil
- 1 bell pepper, sliced
- 4 green onions, sliced
- 2 teaspoons sesame oil
- 1 teaspoon of red pepper flakes

Instructions:

1. Mix dry sherry, coconut amino, garlic and ginger in a bowl. Add chicken and coat well Marinate for 30 minutes.
2. Add about 2 tablespoons water to a deep plate and add zoodles. Cover and microwave for 1 minute. Drain.
3. Preheat 1 tablespoon oil in a skillet over medium heat. Add chicken and cook for about 4 minutes per side. Remove from the pan.
4. Add 1 more tablespoon oil and add bell pepper, cook for 1-2 minutes, stirring frequently.
5. Add the marinade and cook for 1-2 minutes more. Add chicken back to the pan and stir well.
6. Serve chicken on top of zoodles. Top with pepper flakes.

Asian Tuna Cakes

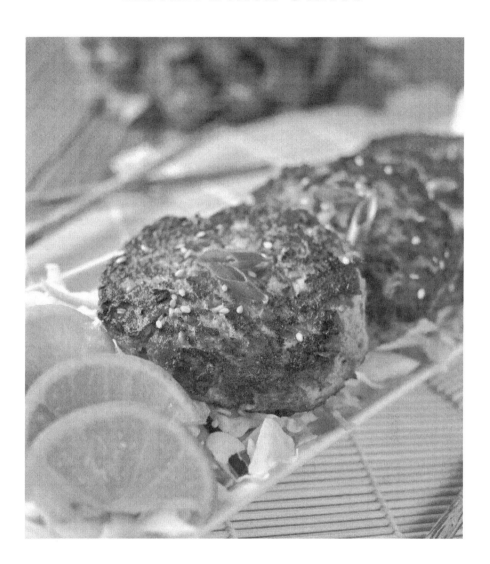

Cooking time: 15 minutes

Servings: 4

Ingredients:

- 7 oz canned tuna, drained
- 2 pastured eggs
- 1 shallot, minced
- 2 garlic cloves, minced
- 2 tablespoons olive oil
- 2 tablespoons fresh parsley, chopped
- 2 tablespoons coconut amino
- 1 teaspoon fresh ginger, grated
- 1 teaspoon toasted sesame seeds
- ¼ teaspoon crushed red pepper flakes
- Sea salt, black pepper, to taste

Instructions:

1. Mix tuna, eggs, shallots, garlic, parsley, coconut amino, ginger, sesame seeds, red pepper flakes, salt and black pepper in a bowl.
2. Form the mixture into patties. Freeze them for 30 minutes.
3. Preheat oil in a skillet over medium heat. Add patties and cook for 3-4 minutes on each side.

Broiled Asian Chicken Thighs

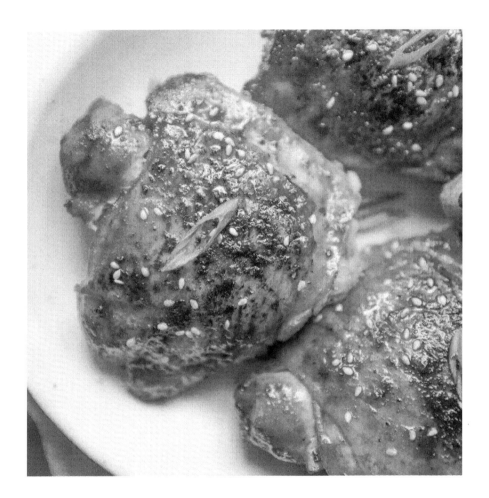

Cooking time: 10 minutes

Servings: 4

Ingredients:

- 1 ½ lbs. Chicken thighs, boneless, skinless
- 2 teaspoons of olive oil
- 2 teaspoons of sesame oil
- 2 ½ teaspoons ketchup or tomato paste
- 2 ½ teaspoons rice wine vinegar
- 1 teaspoon Sriracha sauce
- 1 garlic clove minced
- 2 ½ teaspoons ginger minced
- 1 lime, juiced

Instructions:

1. Mix olive oil, sesame oil, ketchup, vinegar, Sriracha, garlic, ginger and lime juice in a bowl. Add chicken thighs and coat well. Marinate for at least 1 hour.
2. Preheat your broiler. Cover a baking sheet with foil, place chicken on the baking sheet.
3. Broil for 5 minutes per side, 4-6 inches from the broiler. Alternatively, you can cook chicken on a grill.

Meatballs in Coconut Broth

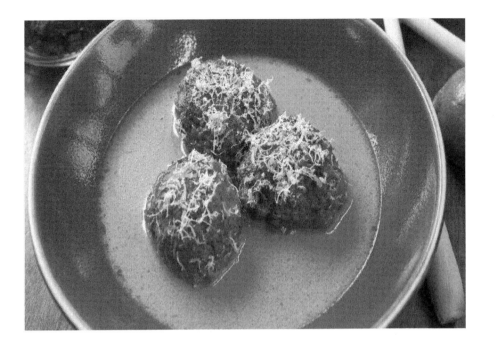

Cooking time: 20 minutes

Servings: 4

Ingredients:

- 1 lb. ground beef
- ½ onion, chopped
- 4 garlic cloves, minced
- 1 tablespoon coconut oil
- ½ cup almond flour
- 2 tablespoons almond milk
- 1 tablespoon pink Himalayan sea salt
- 1 cup coconut milk
- 1 cup chicken or vegetable broth
- 2 teaspoons coriander seeds
- 1 teaspoon turmeric
- 1 teaspoon cinnamon
- 1 teaspoon crushed red pepper
- 1 stalk lemongrass
- 1-inch piece of fresh ginger, grated
- 1 lime, zested

Instructions:

1. Preheat oil in a skillet over medium heat. Add onion and cook for 3-4 minutes. Add garlic and cook for 30 seconds more.
2. Mix almond flour and milk in a bowl. Add salt and flour and milk mixture to the beef. Add the cooked onion and garlic and mix with your hands, until combined.
3. Form the mixture into balls. Add oil to the skillet and preheat well. Arrange the meatballs along the edge of the skillet and leave the center empty.
4. Add coriander, turmeric, cinnamon and red pepper to the center of the skillet. Cook meatballs until brown on all sides.
5. Add coconut milk and broth, stir well. Add lemongrass and ginger. Cook for 3-5 minutes. Serve.

Thai Chicken Green Curry

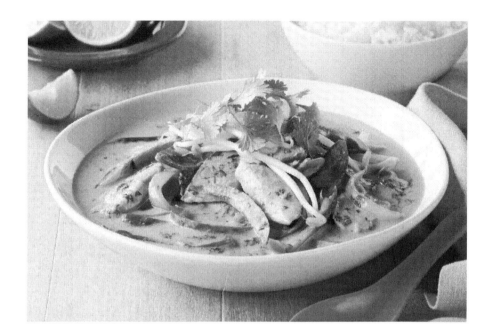

Cooking time: 15 minutes

Servings: 4

Ingredients:

- 1 ½ lbs. chicken breasts, cut into bite-sized pieces
- 1 tablespoon sesame oil
- 2 tablespoons Thai green curry paste
- 1 garlic clove
- 1 ½ cups coconut milk
- ½ cup chicken stock
- 2 lemongrass stalks, chopped
- 1 lime, juiced
- 2 limes, zested
- 1 cup sugar snap peas
- 1 cup bean sprouts
- A handful fresh coriander leaves, for serving

Instructions:

1. Preheat oil in a skillet over medium heat. Add chicken and cook until browned on all sides.
2. Add lemongrass, garlic, curry paste and lime zest to skillet and cook for 2-3 minutes.
3. Add coconut milk, stock and lime juice. Reduce the heat to low, cover the skillet and cook for 10 minutes.
4. Add peas and cook for 2 minutes. Add sprouts and cook for 1 minute more.
5. Serve topped with coriander.

Chicken with Satay Sauce

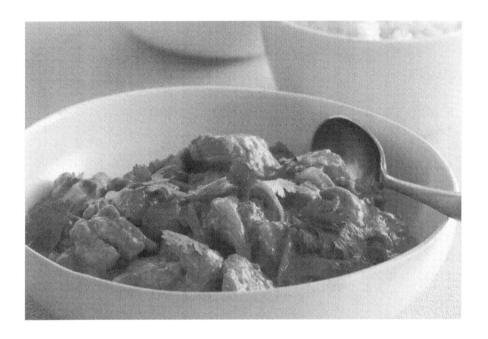

Cooking time: 20 minutes

Servings: 4

Ingredients:

- 1 ½ lbs. chicken thighs, cut into bite-size pieces
- 14 oz coconut milk
- 1 red chili pepper, deseeded and chopped
- 1 garlic clove, chopped
- ¼ cup soy sauce
- 8 tablespoons peanut butter
- 1 tablespoon fresh ginger, minced
- 1 teaspoon turmeric
- 1 tablespoon coriander seed
- 3 tablespoons coconut oil
- Salt, to taste

Instructions:

1. Mix ginger, turmeric, coriander and oil in a bowl. Pour over chicken and marinate for 5-10 minutes.
2. Mix coconut milk, red chili pepper, garlic, soy sauce and peanut butter in a small saucepan. Bring to a boil over low heat, cook for 5-10 minutes until the sauce thickens. Add salt to taste.
3. Preheat oil in a skillet over medium heat. Add chicken and cook for 3-4 minutes. Season with salt and cook for 2-3 minutes on low heat, stirring often.
4. Serve chicken topped with sauce.

Thai Fish with Curry and Coconut

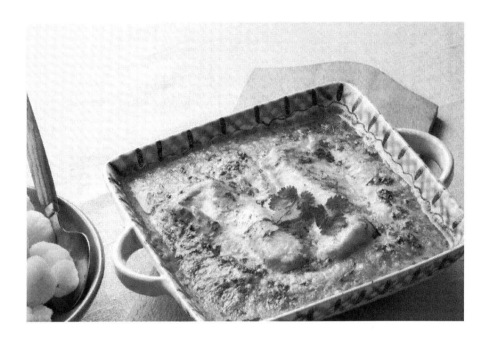

Cooking time: 23 minutes

Servings: 4

Ingredients:

- 1 ½ lbs. white fish, cut into bite-sized pieces
- 2 cups broccoli florets
- 1 tablespoon olive oil
- 4 tablespoons butter
- 2 tablespoons red curry paste
- 1 can (14 oz) coconut cream
- ½ cup fresh cilantro, chopped
- Salt, pepper, to taste

Instructions:

1. Preheat the oven to 400F. Grease a baking dish with olive oil.
2. Place fish into the baking dish. Season with salt and pepper and add 1 tablespoon of butter on top of each fish piece.
3. Mix coconut cream, curry paste and cilantro in a bowl and pour over the fish.
4. Bake for 20 minutes.
5. Boil broccoli florets in lightly salted water for 2-3 minutes. Serve with the fish.

Almond Chili Beef and Cabbage Noodles

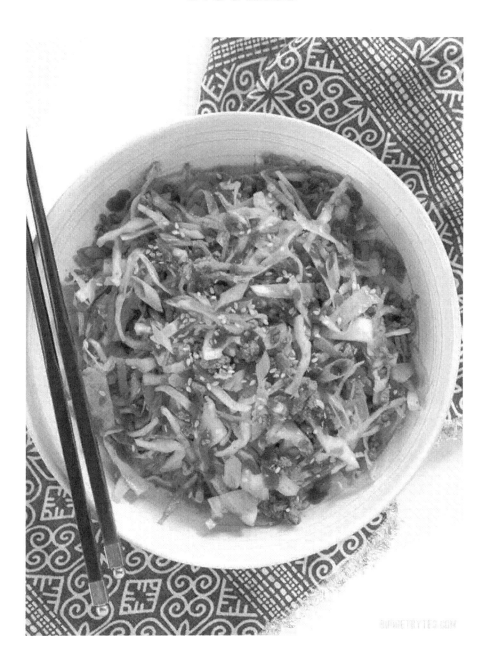

Cooking time: 15 minutes

Servings: 4

Ingredients:

- 1 lb. ground beef
- 1 cabbage head, finely chopped
- 1 tablespoon olive oil
- 6 tablespoons almond butter
- 2 tablespoons coconut vinegar
- 2 tablespoons coconut amino
- 2 tablespoons water
- 2 tablespoons toasted sesame oil
- 2 tablespoons Sriracha sauce
- 10 drops liquid Stevia
- Green Onions, for serving
- Sesame seeds, for serving

Instructions:

1. Add olive oil, ground beef and cabbage to a large pan, spread on the bottom. Cover the pan and cook on medium heat for 10 minutes.
2. Uncover the pan and stir everything for 5 minutes.
3. Mix almond butter, vinegar, coconut amino, water, sesame oil, Sriracha sauce and stevia in a bowl. Pour the sauce over beef and cabbage and mix well to combine.
4. Serve topped with onions and sesame seeds.

Sesame Crusted Chicken Tenders

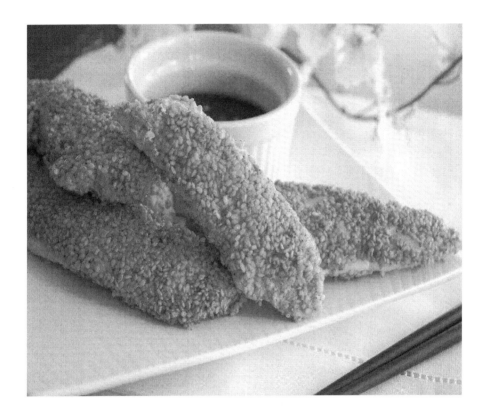

Cooking time: 10 minutes

Servings: 4

Ingredients:

- 1 lb. chicken tenders
- 1 egg white
- ¾ cup sesame seeds
- 2 tablespoons sesame oil + 1 tablespoon
- ¼ cup low-sodium soy sauce
- 2 tablespoons apple cider vinegar
- 1 red Serrano chili, diced
- 1 garlic clove, crushed
- ½ teaspoon ground ginger
- ½ teaspoon of red pepper flakes
- Salt, pepper, to taste

Instructions:

1. Mix soy sauce, vinegar, Serrano chili, garlic, ginger, red pepper flakes and 1 tablespoon sesame oil in a bowl, refrigerate the sauce for 1 hour.
2. Pat dry chicken tenders and season with salt and pepper.
3. Whisk egg white in a bowl. Dip chicken tenders first in egg and then in sesame seeds.
4. Preheat oil in a skillet over medium heat. Add chicken and cook for 4 minutes per side.
5. Serve with sauce.

Low Carb Asian Salmon Stir Fry

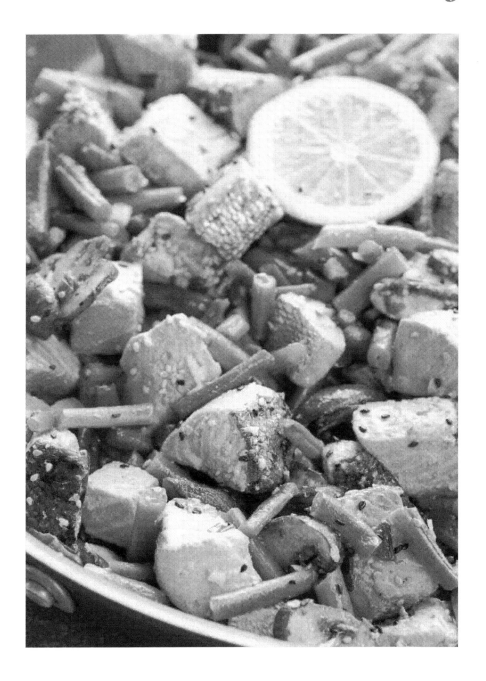

Cooking time: 13 minutes

Servings: 4

Ingredients:

- 1 ½ lbs. Salmon fillets, cubed
- 11 oz green beans, trimmed and chopped
- 2 cups mushrooms, sliced
- 1 tablespoon garlic, crushed
- 1 tablespoon ginger minced
- 3 tablespoons soy sauce
- 2 teaspoons sesame oil
- ½ lemon, juiced
- ¼ cup green onions, chopped
- ½ tablespoon sesame seeds, for serving

Instructions:

1. Mix salmon and 2 tablespoons soy sauce in a bowl. Let marinate for couple of minutes.
2. Preheat 1 teaspoon oil in a skillet over medium heat. Add salmon, half of garlic and ginger and cook for 8-10 minutes, stirring occasionally. Transfer to a plate.
3. Add remaining oil, garlic and ginger, beans, mushrooms and soy sauce, and cook for 5 minutes, stirring often.
4. Return salmon to the pan and add lemon juice, stir well to combine. Serve topped with onions and sesame seeds.

Miso Salmon with Cauliflower Rice

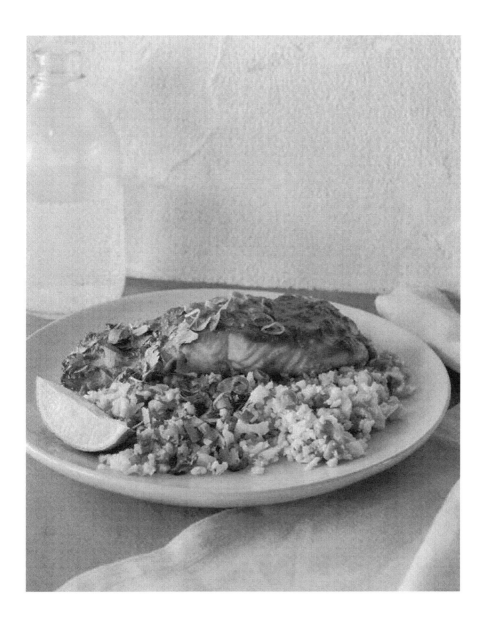

Cooking time: 8 minutes + marinating

Servings: 2

Ingredients:

- 1 lb. salmon fillet, cut into bite-sized pieces
- 2 cups cauliflower rice
- 1 tablespoon soy sauce
- 1 tablespoon butter
- 2 tablespoons miso
- 2 tablespoons Japanese Sake
- 2 teaspoons sweetener of choice
- 1 green onion, chopped

Instructions:

1. Mix miso, Sake and sweetener in a bowl, add salmon and toss well to coat. Marinate in the fridge for at least 8 hours.
2. Preheat the oven to 425F.
3. Pat dry marinated salmon with paper towels. Line a baking sheet with foil, place salmon on the sheet. Bake for 8 minutes.
4. Heat butter in a skillet over medium heat. Add cauliflower rice and cook for 3-5 minutes, stirring frequently.
5. Serve salmon with rice topped with green onion.

Fish with Japanese Mayo Sauce

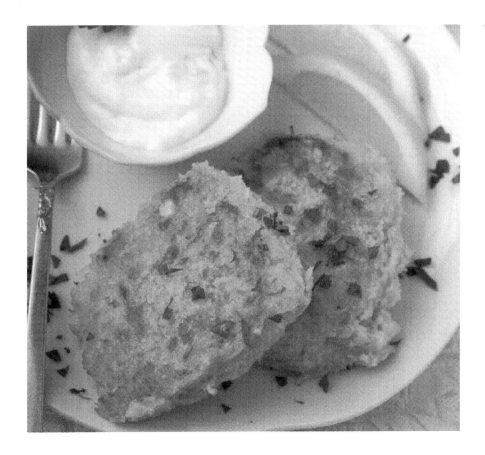

Cooking time: 20 minutes

Servings: 2

Ingredients:

- 1lb white fish fillet
- 1 cup almond flour
- 2 eggs
- 3 ¾ cups unflavored pork rinds
- 4 tablespoons Kewpie Mayo
- 1 teaspoon sweetener of choice
- 1 teaspoon Dijon mustard
- Green onion, chopped
- Salt, pepper, to taste

Instructions:

1. Preheat the oven to 400F. Line a baking sheet with foil, spray with cooking oil.
2. Pat dry the fish with paper towels and sprinkle with salt and pepper from all sides.
3. Add all the pork rinds to a food processor and blend until the texture of breadcrumbs.
4. Beat eggs in one small bowl. Add almond flour to the second bowl and pork rinds to the third bowl.
5. Dip the fish first in flour, then egg and finally in breadcrumbs. Place on a baking sheet.
6. Bake for 10 minutes, turn and cook for 10 minutes more.
7. Mix Kewpie Mayo, sweetener, mustard and green onions in a bowl. Serve the fish with the sauce.

Low Carb Pork Lo Mein

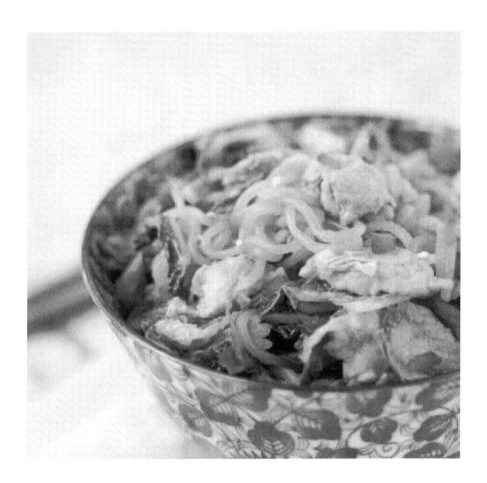

Cooking time: 18 minutes

Servings: 4

Ingredients:

- 1 lb. pork sirloin, sliced
- 16 oz Shiitake noodles
- 2 cups Napa cabbage, shredded
- ½ cup mushrooms, sliced
- 1 tablespoon soy sauce + ½ cup
- 1 tablespoon avocado oil
- 1 cup scallions, sliced
- 2 garlic cloves, sliced
- 1 teaspoon sesame oil
- 1 teaspoon ginger minced
- 2 tablespoons rice wine vinegar
- 1 tablespoon sweetener of choice
- 1 teaspoon Sriracha sauce
- 2 teaspoons hoisin sauce

Instructions:

1. Add noodles to a colander, rinse well and drain.
2. Mix pork, 1 tablespoon soy sauce and marinate for 5-10 minutes.
3. Preheat avocado oil in a skillet over medium heat. Add pork and cook for about 2 minutes. Remove from skillet and set aside.
4. Add mushrooms and cook for 2 minutes, then remove from skillet.
5. Add garlic, scallions and cabbage, cook for 1 minute. Remove from heat and add noodles to skillet, toss well to combine.
6. Mix ½ cup soy sauce, sesame oil, ginger, vinegar, sweetener, Sriracha and hoisin in a bowl. Pour the sauce to the skillet with noodles and heat over medium heat, cook for 2-3 minutes and toss well to coat noodles. Serve.

Matcha Cheesecake

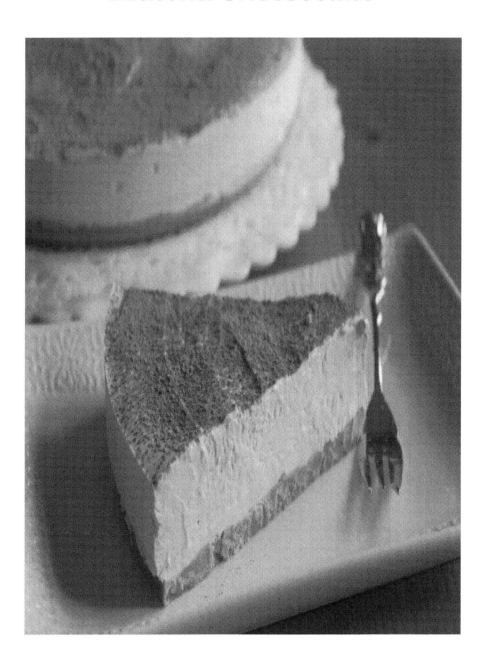

Cooking time: 1 hour 20 minutes

Servings: 10

Ingredients:

- 16 oz cream cheese
- ¾ cup sour cream
- ¾ cup heavy cream
- ½ cup erythritol
- 1 teaspoon Stevia powder
- 1 teaspoon vanilla extract
- 2 tablespoons matcha powder
- 3 eggs

For the Crust:

- ¾ cup almond flour
- ¼ cup pistachios, chopped
- ¼ teaspoon Stevia powder
- 2 tablespoons butter, melted
- 1 teaspoon matcha powder

Instructions:

1. Preheat the oven to 300F.
2. Mix all the ingredients for the Curst in a bowl. Transfer it to a springform pan and press to the bottom, spreading evenly.
3. Bake the crust for 10 minutes.
4. Meanwhile, smooth cream cheese in a bowl with a hand mixer. Add erythritol, stevia and vanilla, mix well until combined.
5. Add sour cream and mix again, then add matcha powder and stir well to combine.
6. Slowly add heavy cream, mixing constantly. Mix until a nice smooth batter is formed.
7. Add one egg at a time, whisk until incorporated. Pour the batter on top of the crust. Place in the oven and cook for about 65-70 minutes.
8. Let rest for 1-2 hours after cooking, then refrigerate overnight.

Coconut Almond Crisps

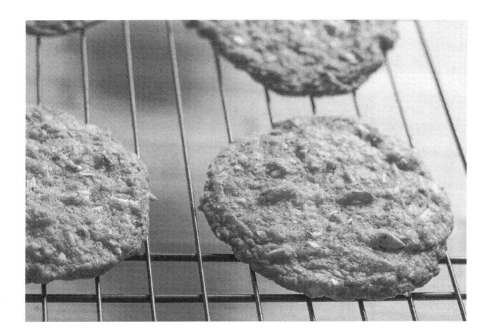

Cooking time: 25 minutes

Servings: 12

Ingredients:

- ¼ cup almond meal
- 6 tablespoons shredded coconut
- ¼ cup butter
- 1/3 cup Swerve sweetener
- 2 teaspoons honey
- ¼ teaspoon flaxseed meal
- ½ teaspoon vanilla extract

Instructions:

1. Preheat the oven to 350F. Line two baking sheets with parchment paper.
2. Mix butter, Swerve and honey in a saucepan, place over medium heat. Cook until sweetener has dissolved, stirring all the time.
3. Remove from heat and add xanthan gum, whisk well to combine. Add almond meal, shredded coconut and vanilla extract.
4. Add about 1 teaspoon of batter on the baking sheet, leaving about 4-inch space between cookies. Press the cookies down to flatten.
5. Bake for 10-12 minutes until cookies are lightly brown. Remove from oven and let cool before serving.

Matcha Pistachio Keto Mug Cake

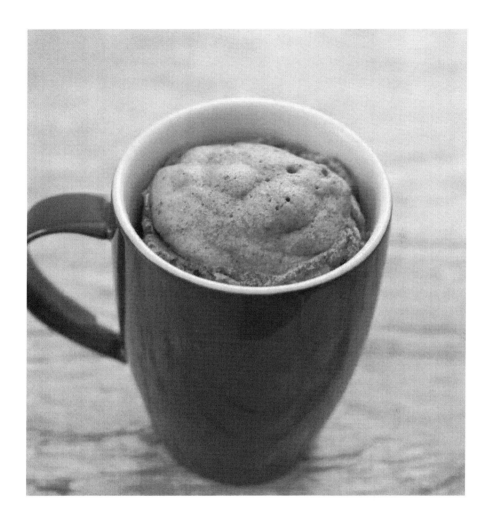

Cooking time: 1 minute

Servings: 2

Ingredients:

- 2 tablespoons almond flour
- 2 tablespoons coconut flour
- 1 egg
- 2 tablespoons erythritol
- 1 tablespoon coconut oil, melted
- 1 tablespoon almond milk
- ½ teaspoon baking powder
- ½ teaspoon matcha powder
- 1 tablespoon pistachios, chopped

Instructions:

1. Whisk together all the ingredients in a bowl. Grease cooking mugs with oil.
2. Transfer the batter to mugs and microwave for 60-90 seconds.
3. **For the oven:** Preheat oven to 350F. Bake mug cake for 10-15 minutes.

Mango Panna Cotta

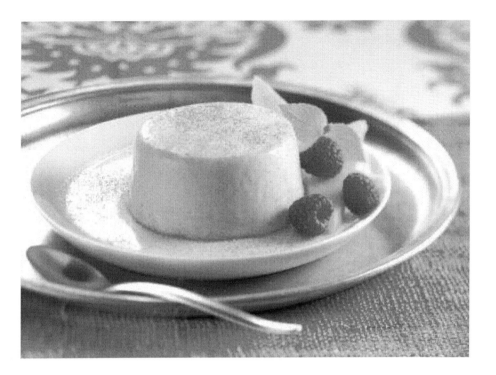

Cooking time: 5 minutes

Servings: 4

Ingredients:

- 1 cup whole milk
- ½ tablespoon unflavored gelatin
- ½ cup heavy whipping cream
- ½ cup mango, diced
- ¼ cup sweetener of choice
- ½ teaspoon ground cardamom

Instructions:

1. Add gelatin to a bowl and pour ½ cup milk on top. Let soak until softened, stirring once.
2. Add cream, mango, sweetener, cardamom and the remaining milk to a food processor or blender. Process until everything is mixed.
3. Pour gelatin and milk mixture to a saucepan and heat over low heat, stirring until gelatin dissolves.
4. Slowly add to the mango mixture and blend again to combine.
5. Pour mixture into cups or glass bowls and refrigerate for 1-2 hours.

Japanese Cotton Cheesecake

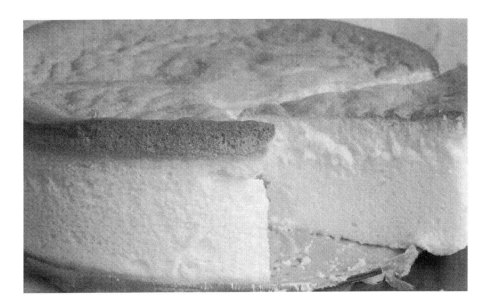

Cooking time: 1 hour

Servings: 4

Ingredients:

- 3 eggs, whites and yolks separated
- 1 cup cream cheese
- ½ cup almond flour
- ½ teaspoon baking powder
- ½ teaspoon Stevia powder
- 1 cup fresh blackberries or other berries of choice, for serving

Instructions:

1. Preheat the oven to 320F. Line a springform pan with parchment paper. Wrap the outer bottom and sides of the pan with foil.
2. Microwave cream cheese for about 40 seconds until soft.
3. Beat egg whites with a hand mixer until stiff peaks form. Beat cream cheese and yolks in a separate bowl.
4. Add half of Stevia, almond flour and baking powder to cream cheese and beat until combined.
5. Sieve the mixture. Sift until it's transferred to a large bowl.
6. Add about 1/3 of the egg white's mixture to the cream cheese batter, stir to incorporate. Add another 1/3 and stir again. Add the last 1/3 and stir well.
7. Pour the batter into the pan and cook for 40 minutes. Turn the temperature down to 285F and cook for 10 minutes more.
8. Let cool completely before serving and top with berries.

Thank You.

I sincerely hope these recipes meet your expectations and assist you on your journey of delicious health.

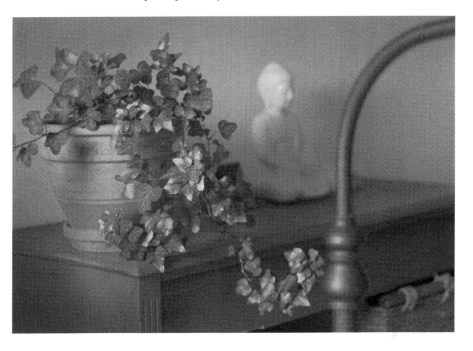

Manufactured by Amazon.ca
Bolton, ON

25128413R00061